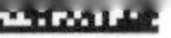

# FROM MANAGING TO CONQUERING DYSHIDROSIS

**Expert Guide To Understanding the Causes, Recognizing Symptoms, Prevention and Embracing Effective Treatments for a Vibrant and Healthy Life**

## DR. DASHIELL DANIEL

## Disclaimer

This book, is intended to provide information and guidance on the subject matter and is not a substitute for professional medical advice, diagnosis, or treatment.

The author, is not a medical professional, and the content presented here is based on research, general knowledge, and expert guidance available at the time of writing.

The information in this book is provided with the understanding that the author and the publisher are not engaged in rendering medical, legal, or other professional services.

Any reliance on the information contained in this book is at the reader's own risk.

While every effort has been made to ensure the accuracy and completeness of the information presented, medical knowledge is constantly evolving, and new research may supersede the content in this book. The author and the publisher make no representations or warranties of any kind, express or implied, about the completeness, accuracy, reliability, suitability, or availability concerning the information, products, services, or related graphics contained in this book.

This book may contain references or mentions of individuals, products, websites, organizations, or other names for informational purposes only.

The author does not own or endorse any such entities mentioned in the book. Any resemblance to actual persons, living or dead, or actual events is purely coincidental.

Readers are encouraged to consult with qualified healthcare professionals for medical advice, diagnosis, and treatment tailored to their specific circumstances.

The author and the publisher disclaim any liability for any loss or risk, personal or otherwise, arising directly or indirectly from the use of the information presented in this book.

By reading this book, the reader acknowledges and agrees to the terms of this disclaimer.

## ABOUT THIS BOOK

"DYSHIDROSIS: Navigating the Path to Dermatological Wellness" is a timely addition to the medical literature that provides a structured exploration of dyshidrosis, from its definition and diagnostic nuances to diverse treatment modalities and holistic approaches. It is a comprehensive guide addressing the nuances of dyshidrosis, a dermatological condition that frequently eludes easy understanding and effective management.

The book's scope goes beyond the management of symptoms; it explores the many facets of dyshidrosis, such as its prevalence, demographics, and the critical distinction between it and other skin conditions. The introduction not only gives a clear definition of the condition, but also emphasizes the significance of actively managing it within the larger landscape of dermatological health.

Each chapter is explained in great detail, starting with an overview of dyshidrosis and moving on to the diagnostic procedure.

Conventional treatment modalities are broken down, providing information on topical steroids, emollients, antihistamines, phototherapy, and oral medications. One of the most important aspects of managing dyshidrosis is lifestyle modifications, which are covered in detail and include identifying triggers, dietary adjustments, and skincare routines.

The book's unique value is found in its thorough coverage of complementary and alternative therapies, such as acupuncture, herbal supplements, and natural remedies. It goes beyond traditional medical interventions and presents a comprehensive framework for overcoming dyshidrosis. The extensive narrative is completed with chapters on prevention strategies, useful advice for everyday living, and a collection of success stories.

DYSHIDROSIS is not just a medical guide; it also discusses the psychological aspects of having dyshidrosis. Chapters on coping mechanisms, how to communicate with healthcare providers effectively, and educational programs highlight the comprehensive approach that is promoted throughout the book. Personal success stories add a relatable element and help people with dyshidrosis feel less alone.

this book is an invaluable tool for anyone attempting to navigate the complexities of dyshidrosis. It is a valuable reference for dermatologists, medical professionals, and anyone interested in learning more about this condition. It provides a path to dermatological wellness and a life free from the limitations of dyshidrosis.

# Introduction

Dyshidrosis is a dermatological condition that causes small, itchy blisters on the palms of the hands and the soles of the feet. It is also referred to as dyshidrotic eczema or pompholyx. Dyshidrosis can be chronic and recurrent, greatly affecting the quality of life for those who experience it. Although it is a common condition, effective management strategies are not always well understood or widely disseminated.

The purpose of this book is to thoroughly examine the definition, etiology, and different management strategies for individuals who suffer from this difficult condition.

## What Dyshidrosis Means

Dyshidrosis is a rare kind of dermatology that usually appears as tiny, fluid-filled blisters on the palms of the hands and soles of the feet.

These blisters are very itchy and can cause redness, swelling, and skin fissuring. The term "dyshidrosis" is a bit misleading because it refers to a type of eczema, specifically dyshidrotic eczema, for which there is no known cause.

The precise etiology entails a complex interaction between a person's genetic predisposition, environmental factors, and immune system responses. Knowing the subtle definition of dyshidrosis paves the way for a deeper investigation of its treatment approaches.

## The Value Of Taking Care Of Dyshidrosis

Dyshidrosis management is more than just treating the physical symptoms. People who live with the condition frequently feel that it has a significant negative impact on their emotional and physical well-being. The constant pain, itching, and concerns about appearance can result in a reduced quality of life. Because dyshidrosis is a chronic condition, it can also cause social and occupational difficulties, which emphasizes the need for comprehensive treatment. Taking care of the condition as a whole not only helps to reduce the physical symptoms but also promotes positive psychological and social aspects.

## The Book's Scope

This book covers a wide range of topics related to dyshidrosis and offers a thorough reference for medical professionals as well as individuals with the condition. From a clinical standpoint, the book will investigate the different diagnostic criteria used to identify dyshidrosis, highlighting the difficulties in correctly diagnosing this dermatological condition. Additionally, it will delve into the pathophysiology of dyshidrosis, taking into account genetic predispositions, immune system dysregulation, and environmental triggers.

Finally, the book will critically examine treatment modalities, from topical corticosteroids to novel therapeutic approaches, with a focus on evidence-based practices.

Apart from the clinical setting, the book will delve into the psychosocial implications of dyshidrosis, clarifying the ways in which the disorder can influence mental health, self-worth, and interpersonal connections. Coping mechanisms for managing the psychological effects of dyshidrosis will be deliberated, recognizing the significance of a multidisciplinary approach to treatment. Furthermore, the book will cover preventive measures, lifestyle adjustments, and current research in the domain, offering readers a prospective outlook on the dynamic field of dyshidrosis management.

Finally, this book attempts to disentangle the complexity of dyshidrosis by providing a thorough manual for medical professionals, researchers, and those impacted by this dermatological issue. By exploring the meaning, significance of treatment, and breadth of dyshidrosis, it hopes to close the gap between scientific knowledge and useful approaches for managing and overcoming this frequently bewildering ailment.

# CHAPTER ONE
# COMPREHENDING DYSHIDROSIS

The dermatological condition dyshidrosis, also called dyshidrotic eczema or pompholyx, is typified by the formation of small, painful blisters on the hands and feet. The blisters are frequently accompanied by redness, swelling, and extreme itching, making it a distressing condition. The term "dyshidrosis" has an etymological connection to sweating, but the exact cause of the condition is unknown. It is thought that a combination of immune responses, environmental factors, and genetic predispositions play a role in the manifestation of dyshidrosis.

## Indications And Features

People who have dyshidrosis frequently develop small, fluid-filled blisters on the palms of their hands, fingers, and the bottoms of their feet.

These blisters can be extremely itchy and uncomfortable, which can lead to scratching and other complications. The skin surrounding the blisters can turn red and swollen, and in extreme circumstances, the blisters can burst, causing the skin to peel and crack. Dyshidrosis patients' quality of life can be greatly reduced by the constant itching and discomfort that come with the condition, as daily tasks involving the use of hands and feet become difficult.

# Reasons And Initiators

Though the exact causes of dyshidrosis are still unknown, a number of factors are thought to play a role in its development. Genetics is one of the main factors, as people who have a family history of eczema or other allergic conditions may be more susceptible to dyshidrosis.

Environmental factors include exposure to chemicals, metals, and allergens, which can cause flare-ups of the condition; stress is another potential trigger, as it can affect the immune system and cause the symptoms of dyshidrosis to appear or worsen. Individuals with atopic dermatitis or other allergic conditions may also be more susceptible to dyshidrosis.

# Recognizing Dyshidrosis Differentially From Other Skin Conditions

Proper differentiation is essential for developing an appropriate treatment plan; this emphasizes the importance of consulting a dermatologist for a thorough evaluation. Dyshidrosis shares similarities with a number of other skin conditions, making accurate diagnosis crucial for effective management. Conditions like psoriasis, contact dermatitis, and fungal infections can manifest with blistering and itching, potentially leading to misdiagnosis. For example, contact dermatitis can result from exposure to irritants or allergens and can present with similar blistering on the hands and feet.

## Demographics And Prevalence

Dyshidrosis is a condition with a variable prevalence that affects people of all ages and ethnicities. Although it can occur at any time in life, it is most commonly observed in adults under 40. Women appear to be more likely than men to have the condition, with some studies suggesting that women are more likely than men.

People who have a personal or family history of eczema, hay fever, or asthma may also be more likely to develop dyshidrosis. Research on the effects of geography and environmental factors on prevalence is still being conducted. These include differences in climate, humidity, and exposure to potential triggers that may affect the occurrence and severity of dyshidrotic eczema in various populations.

comprehending dyshidrosis entails identifying its signs and features, investigating possible causes and triggers, separating it from other skin conditions, and taking into account its prevalence and demographics.

By having a thorough understanding of these elements, medical practitioners can create specialized plans to treat and lessen dyshidrosis sufferers' symptoms, ultimately enhancing their quality of life.

# CHAPTER TWO
# DYSHIDROSIS DIAGNOSIS

Dyshidrosis, also called dyshidrotic eczema or pompholyx, is a dermatological condition that causes small, itchy blisters to form on the palms of the hands and the soles of the feet. It is important to recognize the symptoms of dyshidrosis in order to make an accurate diagnosis. The first sign of the condition is typically the appearance of tiny, deep-seated vesicles filled with clear fluid, often accompanied by redness and intense itching. These blisters may group together, forming patches that cause discomfort and distress to the affected individuals. Additionally, the condition can worsen by causing fissures, scaling, and peeling of the skin. Patients may also notice a cyclical pattern of flare-ups followed by periods of remission.

Seeking Professional Diagnosis: Due to the variable nature of skin conditions and the possibility of misidentification, it is essential for those exhibiting symptoms suggestive of dyshidrosis to seek professional diagnosis. Dermatologists, as experts in skin disorders, are essential in correctly diagnosing and treating dyshidrosis. During the diagnostic process, a thorough examination of the affected areas is usually combined with a thorough medical history. The healthcare provider may ask about the onset, duration, and triggers of symptoms, as well as any pertinent family or personal medical history. Professional diagnosis not only helps rule out other dermatological conditions with similar presentations but also makes it possible to formulate an efficient treatment plan.

Diagnostic Tests and Procedures: Dermatologists may suggest diagnostic tests and procedures to confirm the diagnosis of dyshidrosis in situations where the clinical presentation is unclear or additional evidence is required. Patch testing, a widely used technique in dermatology, can be used to identify potential allergens causing the skin reaction. This involves applying small amounts of different substances to the skin and monitoring for any negative reactions. Skin biopsies can also be carried out to examine tissue samples under a microscope, which can provide insight into the cellular changes characteristic of dyshidrosis. Dermoscopy, a non-invasive technique that involves using a handheld device to magnify and visualize the skin's surface, may also be utilized to support the diagnosis of dyshidrosis.

# CHAPTER THREE
# CONVENTIONAL THERAPY METHODS

The skin condition dyshidrosis, also called dyshidrotic eczema or pompholyx, is characterized by the formation of small, itchy blisters on the hands and feet. The condition is treated with a variety of conventional strategies, each of which focuses on a different aspect of the condition.

The goal of traditional treatment for dyshidrosis is to minimize symptoms and avoid recurrence.

## Topical Medication

One of the most important tools in the treatment of dyshidrosis is topical steroids. These anti-inflammatory agents work by suppressing the immune response and reducing skin inflammation, which helps to relieve itching and stop blisters from forming. In the clinical setting, doctors typically prescribe mid-potency to high-potency topical steroids for affected areas.

Although these agents are effective, long-term use of them can cause side effects like skin thinning and discoloration, so careful and monitored application is required. Follow-up visits with healthcare providers are essential to monitor progress and make necessary treatment adjustments.

# Moisturizers And Emollients

The use of moisturizers and emollients is essential for managing dyshidrosis because they keep the skin hydrated and prevent it from becoming too dry. Applying these products on a regular basis also helps to create a protective barrier that lowers the likelihood of flare-ups. Ceramide, fatty acid, and cholesterol containing emollients is especially helpful because it mimics the natural skin barrier. Patients should use these products often, especially after taking a bath to lock in moisture.

### Inhibitors of histamine

As an adjuvant treatment for dyshidrosis, antihistamines block the histamine release that causes itching. They may not prevent blisters from forming, but they do alleviate the discomfort that comes with the condition. Non-drowsy antihistamines, like cetirizine or loratadine, are often prescribed to reduce the effect on daily activities. Nevertheless, each patient responds differently to these medications, so doctors may need to modify the dosage or suggest other treatments.

# Photodynamic Therapy

The management of dyshidrosis has been shown to benefit from phototherapy, which involves exposure to ultraviolet (UV) light. UVB therapy, in particular, is frequently used to suppress inflammation and lessen the severity of symptoms. Phototherapy is usually administered under the supervision of healthcare professionals, and the length and intensity of treatment are customized to meet the needs of each patient.

Frequent monitoring is necessary to monitor progress and minimize potential side effects.

# Oral Drugs

When topical treatments and other conventional approaches are insufficient, oral medications are considered. Systemic corticosteroids are prescribed for short periods of time to control acute flare-ups; however, long-term use of these drugs is generally avoided due to the risk of systemic side effects. Immunosuppressive drugs such as methotrexate or cyclosporine are occasionally considered, especially in cases of severe dyshidrosis that is resistant to other treatments. The decision to use oral medications requires careful consideration of the risks and benefits, and close monitoring is essential to manage any potential adverse effects.

To sum up, the conventional methods of treating dyshidrosis involve an all-encompassing approach that addresses inflammation, dehydration, itching, and immune modulation. Each of these approaches has a specific function in the management of this difficult skin condition, and medical professionals customize treatment regimens based on each patient's needs and response. Frequent check-ups and monitoring are essential elements of managing dyshidrosis effectively, guaranteeing the best possible results while reducing the possibility of adverse effects.

# CHAPTER FOUR
# CHANGES IN LIFESTYLE

## Recognizing Triggers

A person's ability to manage and prevent dyshidrosis, a skin condition marked by tiny, itchy blisters on the hands and feet, depends on their ability to identify triggers. Allergens are known to cause dyshidrotic eczema, so people should get tested for them in order to determine which specific substances might make their condition worse. Common allergens include certain metals, fragrances, and preservatives found in personal care products. Environmental factors, such as exposure to extreme temperatures or humidity, can also cause flare-ups.

## Modifications To Diet

Dietary changes can significantly affect the management of dyshidrosis. Certain foods can aggravate symptoms and cause inflammation. People with dyshidrotic eczema should think about adopting an anti-inflammatory diet that includes foods high in omega-3 fatty acids, antioxidants, and vitamins. These foods can help with inflammation reduction and promote overall skin health. Moreover, identifying and removing potential food allergens through an elimination diet can be helpful. Consulting with a medical professional or registered dietitian can offer individualized advice to create a diet plan that is specific to each person's needs and triggers.

## Skincare Routines

For those with dyshidrotic eczema, good skincare practices are critical. It's a delicate balance to maintain proper hygiene without aggravating skin irritation. The use of mild, fragrance-free cleansers and avoiding harsh soaps helps prevent further skin dryness. Moisturization is an important part of skincare; people should use hypoallergenic and fragrance-free moisturizers to keep the skin hydrated. Emollients can form a protective barrier on a regular basis, lowering the risk of flare-ups. Lastly, knowing when to bathe in warm water instead of hot water is critical for preventing skin dehydration.

## Options For Clothes And Fabrics

Clothing and fabric choices have a big influence on how well people manage their dyshidrosis. People should choose loose-fitting, breathable fabrics like cotton to help the skin breathe. Tight or synthetic clothing can trap moisture and make symptoms worse. People should avoid wearing wool and other irritating fabrics directly on areas of their skin that are already inflamed. People should also choose clothing made of natural, soft materials to help the healing process. Finally, people should pay attention to laundry detergents and make sure they are free of harsh chemicals or fragrances.

To sum up, lifestyle adjustments are critical to managing dyshidrosis. Knowing what triggers to avoid, such as allergens and environmental factors, enables people to make educated decisions about their everyday activities and environment.

Dietary adjustments, which emphasize anti-inflammatory foods and the removal of potential allergens, improve overall skin health. Skincare routines, which emphasize gentle cleansing and adequate moisturization, are critical to preventing exacerbations. Carefully chosen clothing and fabrics can also greatly reduce discomfort and aid in the healing process for people with dyshidrotic eczema. Putting these lifestyle adjustments into practice holistically can enable people to better manage and lessen the effects of dyshidrotic eczema.

# CHAPTER FIVE
# COMPLEMENTARY AND ALTERNATIVE THERAPIES
## Natural Solutions

Aloe Vera: For centuries, people seeking natural remedies have used Aloe Vera for a variety of skin conditions, including dyshidrosis. The gel extracted from Aloe Vera leaves contains bioactive compounds with anti-inflammatory and moisturizing effects. When applied topically, Aloe Vera may help soothe the irritated and inflamed skin associated with dyshidrosis. Its ability to accelerate wound healing and reduce itching makes it a popular choice. It's important to note, though, that although Aloe Vera can offer relief, its effectiveness may differ from person to person and more research is required to determine its precise function in dyshidrosis management.

Apple Cider Vinegar (ACV): Another natural remedy that has gained popularity in the management of dyshidrosis is ACV. It is thought to have antimicrobial and anti-inflammatory properties, which may help alleviate symptoms associated with this skin condition. Diluted ACV can be applied topically or added to bathwater for a soak.

Since ACV is acidic, it may help restore the pH balance of the skin and create an environment that is less conducive to the development of blisters. However, it is important to use caution when using undiluted ACV because it can be harsh on the skin. Additionally, there is not enough scientific evidence to support the efficacy of ACV in treating dyshidrosis, requiring further research to confirm its therapeutic potential.

Oatmeal Baths: Oatmeal baths have been used for many years to treat a variety of skin conditions, including dyshidrosis. Colloidal oatmeal, which is made of finely ground oats that dissolve into a milky dispersion when poured into water, is well-known for its anti-inflammatory and skin-soothing qualities. Soaking in an oatmeal bath can help relieve itching, reduce inflammation, and improve overall skin comfort.

The fine oat particles form a protective layer on the skin, assisting in moisture retention. Although oatmeal baths are generally thought to be safe and well-tolerated, people who have oat allergies should proceed with caution.

Acupuncture: Based in traditional Chinese medicine, acupuncture uses thin needles inserted into specific body points to stimulate energy flow and restore balance. Some people with dyshidrosis use acupuncture as a complementary therapy to reduce symptoms. Proponents claim that acupuncture can modulate immune system and reduce inflammation, helping to manage skin conditions. There is limited research supporting acupuncture's potential benefits, but it is not conclusive when it comes to treating dyshidrosis. Research gaps remain, and more thorough clinical trials are required to ascertain the genuine efficacy of acupuncture as an adjunctive treatment for this dermatological condition.

Herbal Supplements: The use of herbal supplements to treat dyshidrosis has generated interest in the field of complementary medicine. A number of herbs, including burdock root, calendula, and turmeric, are thought to have immune-modulating and anti-inflammatory properties. These supplements are meant to promote skin health in general and relieve the symptoms of dyshidrosis. However, there is a lack of scientific evidence to support the effectiveness of herbal supplements in treating dyshidrosis, and patients should exercise caution as there may be medication interactions or allergic reactions. Patients should speak with healthcare providers before incorporating herbal supplements into their treatment plan.

Mind-Body Techniques: Mind-body techniques, which include mindfulness, meditation, and guided imagery, have been recognized for their potential to help manage a variety of health conditions, including dermatological disorders like dyshidrosis. Since stress is thought to be a potential cause of flare-ups for dyshidrosis, mind-body techniques work to reduce stress and promote relaxation.

By doing so, people may feel less stressed, which may help to improve the symptoms of dyshidrosis. Although preliminary research indicates that mind-body techniques may be beneficial for some skin conditions, more research is required to clarify the precise effects of mind-body techniques on dyshidrosis and to establish standard protocols for their incorporation into treatment regimens.

In conclusion, alternative and complementary therapies offer a diverse array of options for individuals seeking additional avenues for managing dyshidrosis. Natural remedies such as Aloe Vera, Apple Cider Vinegar, and oatmeal baths showcase the potential benefits of harnessing the healing properties of botanical and naturally derived substances. Acupuncture and herbal supplements, rooted in traditional medicine practices, introduce alternative approaches that warrant further investigation to solidify their place in dyshidrosis management.

Additionally, mind-body techniques emphasize the interconnectedness of mental and physical well-being, suggesting that stress reduction may play a pivotal role in ameliorating dyshidrosis symptoms. It is imperative for individuals considering these therapies to approach them with an informed mindset, understanding that while anecdotal evidence exists, rigorous scientific scrutiny is essential for establishing their efficacy and safety in the context of dyshidrosis.

Collaborative efforts between healthcare professionals, researchers, and individuals seeking relief from dyshidrosis are crucial for advancing our understanding of these alternative approaches and integrating them into comprehensive and evidence-based treatment strategies.

# CHAPTER SIX
# OVERCOMING DYSHIDROSIS HOLISTICALLY
## Integrative Methods

Dyshidrosis, a skin condition characterized by the development of small, itchy blisters on the hands and feet, necessitates a comprehensive and integrative approach for effective management. Integrative approaches involve combining traditional medical treatments with complementary and alternative therapies to address the multifaceted nature of the condition. Dermatological interventions such as topical corticosteroids or immunomodulators may be coupled with holistic treatments like dietary modifications and herbal supplements.

This integrative strategy aims to not only alleviate the symptoms but also target the underlying factors contributing to dyshidrosis. By considering the interplay of genetic, environmental, and lifestyle factors, individuals can tailor an integrative plan that suits their unique needs. This approach acknowledges the importance of a holistic perspective in managing dyshidrosis, recognizing that the condition is not solely a superficial skin issue but may be influenced by various internal and external elements.

## The Value Of Stress Reduction

The holistic approach to treating dyshidrosis necessitates the management of stress because it has been shown to be a trigger and aggravating factor for the condition. Given the complex relationship between the nervous system and the skin, chronic stress can cause immune dysregulation and inflammatory responses, which can lead to the onset or worsening of dyshidrosis symptoms. Including stress reduction techniques like yoga, deep breathing exercises, and mindfulness meditation in the holistic treatment plan can have a positive effect on the health of the skin. Additionally, psychotherapeutic interventions like cognitive-behavioral therapy may assist individuals in coping with stressors in a way that will lessen the impact on their skin.

## Harmonizing Mental And Physical Health

Achieving a balance between physical and mental well-being is imperative in the holistic management of dyshidrosis. Physical health encompasses lifestyle factors such as diet, exercise, and sleep, which can significantly influence the skin's condition. Adopting an anti-inflammatory diet rich in antioxidants, omega-3 fatty acids, and vitamins can support the body's immune response and promote skin health. Regular exercise not only contributes to overall well-being but also aids in stress reduction, indirectly benefiting dyshidrosis management. Adequate sleep is crucial for skin repair and regeneration, and disruptions in sleep patterns can adversely affect the skin's barrier function. Concurrently, addressing mental well-being involves managing stress, anxiety, and depression, as these emotional states can impact the immune system and exacerbate dyshidrosis symptoms. Integrating strategies for both physical and mental well-being into the holistic approach acknowledges the interconnectedness of these aspects in maintaining skin health.

## Putting Up A Support Structure

The holistic conquest of dyshidrosis extends beyond individual efforts and emphasizes the importance of establishing a robust support system. Living with a chronic skin condition can be emotionally challenging, and having a support network can provide emotional, practical, and informational assistance. This support system may include family members, friends, healthcare professionals, and even online communities where individuals can share experiences and insights. Effective communication with healthcare providers ensures that treatment plans are tailored to individual needs and concerns.

Additionally, emotional support from friends and family can alleviate the psychological burden associated with dyshidrosis. Building a strong support system fosters resilience and empowers individuals to navigate the challenges of living with dyshidrosis more effectively. The collective efforts of healthcare professionals, social support networks, and individual commitment contribute to a holistic approach that addresses the physical, emotional, and social dimensions of dyshidrosis management.

treating dyshidrosis holistically entails an integrative approach that takes into account the interaction of multiple factors that influence the condition. Combining conventional medical treatments with complementary therapies, such as stress management techniques and lifestyle adjustments, guarantees a comprehensive strategy. Stress management is an essential component, considering its effect on immune function and inflammatory responses. It is crucial to balance physical and mental well-being, realizing the interdependence of lifestyle factors, emotional states, and skin health. Creating a strong support network further strengthens the holistic approach, recognizing the emotional struggles associated with living with dyshidrosis.

# CHAPTER SEVEN
## STRATEGIES FOR PREVENTION
### Finding And Steering Clear Of Triggers

When it comes to managing dyshidrosis, one of the most important aspects of prevention is identifying and avoiding triggers. Dyshidrosis is typified by the development of tiny, itchy blisters on the palms, fingers, and soles of the feet, and it is frequently sensitive to certain triggers. Finding these triggers is critical for people who want to prevent recurrent outbreaks. Common triggers include exposure to nickel, specific chemicals, or environmental factors like hot and humid conditions.

Thorough dermatological assessments, including patch testing, can help identify individual allergens. Once identified, people can take proactive steps to avoid these triggers, which will lower the chance of developing dyshidrotic flare-ups.

## Practices For Skincare And Hygiene

The prevention of dyshidrosis is largely dependent on good skincare and hygiene practices.

The condition is made worse by factors like excessive moisture, poor hygiene, and skin irritation, so people who are prone to dyshidrotic eczema need to follow a strict skincare routine.

This includes regular but gentle cleansing with mild, fragrance-free soaps to prevent skin irritation; moisturizing is essential, but the choice of moisturizers is important; choosing hypoallergenic and fragrance-free formulations can help to maintain skin health; additionally, people should limit their time spent in the water, as excessive moisture can cause dyshidrotic episodes; wearing gloves when engaging in activities that may irritate the skin

# Guidelines For Nutrition In Prevention

Nutritional guidelines stand as an often-overlooked but significant aspect in the prevention of dyshidrosis.

Research suggests a potential link between diet and the occurrence of eczematous conditions, including dyshidrosis.

Individuals may benefit from adopting an anti-inflammatory diet rich in omega-3 fatty acids, found in sources like fatty fish and flaxseeds, to mitigate inflammatory responses associated with dyshidrotic eczema. Conversely, certain foods, such as dairy, gluten, and artificial additives, may act as triggers for some individuals and should be approached with caution.

Adequate hydration is fundamental for overall skin health, and individuals prone to dyshidrosis should ensure sufficient water intake. Collaborating with healthcare professionals, including dermatologists and nutritionists, can facilitate the development of personalized nutritional strategies to prevent dyshidrotic outbreaks. In summary, recognizing the interplay between nutrition and dyshidrosis opens avenues for proactive prevention through dietary interventions tailored to individual needs.

In summary, managing dyshidrosis requires a multimodal approach, whereby prevention strategies are critical. By recognizing and avoiding triggers, which include allergens and environmental factors, people can take proactive steps to mitigate the onset of dyshidrotic eczema. At the same time, implementing effective skincare and hygiene practices helps to protect the skin from outside irritants and maintain optimal skin health. The incorporation of nutritional guidelines further enhances these strategies by acknowledging the potential influence of diet on inflammatory responses linked to dyshidrosis.

By committing to a thorough preventive regimen that includes these ideas, people can drastically reduce the frequency and severity of their dyshidrotic eczema.

# CHAPTER EIGHT
# HANDYSHIDROSIS: UTILITIVE ADVICE

Dyshidrosis is a dermatological condition that causes small, itchy blisters on the hands and feet. Coping strategies are essential for managing the challenges associated with this condition.

Keeping hands and feet clean can help prevent flare-ups. Moisturizing on a regular basis, especially with emollients that contain hypoallergenic ingredients, can relieve dryness and stop blisters from developing. Using cool compresses and avoiding triggers like stress and certain allergens can also help.

Finally, investigating stress-reduction practices like yoga and meditation may be a useful addition to conventional treatments for patients with dyshidrosis.

# Interacting With Healthcare Professionals

For patients with dyshidrosis, it is critical to establish effective communication with healthcare providers. By accurately communicating the nature and severity of symptoms, patients can help healthcare professionals formulate appropriate treatment plans. Patients should also actively engage in discussions about potential triggers, lifestyle factors, and any coexisting conditions, as these details can significantly influence the course of treatment. Finally, people should ask about new therapeutic options and take part in shared decision-making to ensure that their preferences and concerns are taken into consideration in the development of a comprehensive care plan.

# Teaching Individuals About Dyshidrosis

It is imperative that people learn about Dyshidrosis in order to create a supportive and understanding community.

Through accurate information about the condition, people can eliminate stigma and dispel misconceptions. Personal experiences can be shared through social media or events in the community in order to humanize the condition and draw attention to the difficulties faced by those who live with Dyshidrosis. Working together with advocacy groups and healthcare professionals can also help develop educational materials, such as pamphlets or online resources, that effectively spread trustworthy information about Dyshidrosis. Increased awareness benefits those who are affected but also encourages empathy and inclusivity in society.

# CHAPTER NINE
# TRIUMPHANT NARRATIVES

Dyshidrosis is a skin condition that causes small, itchy blisters to appear on the hands and feet. While many people have struggled with this skin condition, there are many success stories that provide insight into strategies that work and victories over this dermatological condition. Personal accounts of people who have overcome dyshidrosis highlight the fortitude and tenacity of those who have faced this condition and often highlight the various approaches that people have used to manage and ultimately overcome their symptoms. These narratives, which range from medical interventions to lifestyle modifications, highlight the significance of a multifaceted strategy in the fight against dyshidrosis.

In these first-person narratives, patients often emphasize how important medical professionals were in helping them overcome their dyshidrosis. Dermatologists, allergists, and other specialists work with patients to create customized treatment regimens that target the unique triggers and symptoms of dyshidrotic eczema. Comprehensive consultations, diagnostic evaluations, and continued support are all important components of the success stories that come out of the dyshidrosis community. Finally, these stories frequently highlight the importance of patience and perseverance, since managing and overcoming dyshidrosis is frequently a gradual and evolving journey.

A recurrent theme in success stories is the investigation of complementary therapies and holistic approaches. People discuss how dietary adjustments, stress management methods, and alternative therapies have helped them feel better. This holistic viewpoint represents an increasing understanding of the relationship between physical and mental health in the context of dyshidrosis. Success stories serve as invaluable resources for those who are living with the condition as well as for medical professionals looking for new and effective management techniques.

# Individual Testimonials Of Overcoming Dyshidrosis

Personal narratives about overcoming dyshidrosis provide a nuanced understanding of the obstacles people encounter and the various tactics they use to regain control over their skin health.

These narratives typically start at the earliest stages of the disease, describing the irritation and discomfort people feel as blisters form and worsen. The journey continues as people work their way through the maze of possible triggers, looking for solutions and solace. People also talk about the emotional toll dyshidrosis takes on their lives, illuminating how visible skin manifestations affect their self-esteem and day-to-day activities.

As the story goes on, patients talk about their experiences with medical professionals who are essential in the diagnosis and management of dyshidrosis.

Dermatologists perform comprehensive examinations, carry out diagnostic tests, and work with patients to create customized treatment plans. The success stories demonstrate the value of a strong doctor-patient relationship in the fight against dyshidrosis. Topical and systemic medications are frequently included in treatment plans, and patients talk about the relief and improvements they have experienced as a result.

In addition to medical treatments, individual narratives explore lifestyle adjustments made to cope with dyshidrosis. Common themes include dietary adjustments, stress management strategies, and the identification of environmental triggers.

Trial and error experiences are shared by participants, highlighting the flexibility needed to manage the intricacies of dyshidrotic eczema.

The tenacity of these narratives adds to the overall theme of empowerment, as participants not only overcome their physical symptoms but also regain control over their lives.

## Overcoming Obstacles And Rejoicing In Success

Overcoming challenges is a recurrent theme that emphasizes the determination required to navigate the complexities of managing dyshidrosis.

These challenges include the trial and error process of identifying triggers, coping with flare-ups, and adapting to the dynamic nature of the condition. Personal accounts frequently delve into the obstacles faced along the way.

From the initial misdiagnoses to the frustration of finding effective treatments, individuals recount the hurdles that tested their resilience.

Victories in the context of dyshidrosis go beyond the simple relief of symptoms. People talk about times when they have triumphed over the psychological effects of the condition, emphasizing the role that mental health plays in the journey as a whole. Victories include confidence that has been restored, a better quality of life, and a refreshed sense of self. People talk about the happiness and relief they feel when they see a noticeable decrease in blistering, itching, and discomfort.

Additionally, overcoming obstacles and acknowledging successes also pertain to social and emotional well-being. People discuss how to talk about their condition with friends, family, and coworkers in a way that promotes understanding and support.

These stories encourage others to continue on their own paths and remind them that living with dyshidrosis involves more than just controlling its physical symptoms; it also involves building resilience and adopting a holistic perspective on health.

# SUMMARY

the journey to conquer dyshidrosis is complex and involves personal stories, overcoming obstacles, and celebrating successes.

Success stories are rays of hope that show the variety of approaches people take to managing and conquering this dermatological challenge. They also underscore the critical role that healthcare providers play, the value of teamwork, and the efficacy of holistic strategies in managing dyshidrosis.

Individual narratives offer a close-up view of the difficulties people encounter, ranging from the first signs of symptoms to the psychological impact of outwardly apparent skin manifestations.

The cooperative efforts of medical staff and patients are essential to the successes reported in these accounts, highlighting the importance of a customized and patient-focused approach. Medications, dietary changes, and complementary therapies all add to the comprehensive outlook that is revealed by these stories.

The theme of conquering dyshidrosis revolves around overcoming obstacles, which include misdiagnosis trials, treatment failure frustration, and the resilience needed to work through the condition's complexities. Celebrating successes goes beyond simply addressing physical symptoms; they also include mental health improvements, confidence gains, and a sense of empowerment. Victories are social as well as personal, as people share strategies for communicating and promoting understanding with their communities.

These components weave together to form a narrative of empowerment, resilience, and adaptability in the grand scheme of conquering dyshidrosis. Success stories offer motivation to those who are coping with the disease by offering a glimpse into strategies that work and encouraging optimism.

The shared experiences of personal narratives deepen our comprehension of the difficulties faced by people with dyshidrosis and the various ways people overcome hardship.

As the story of conquering dyshidrosis unfolds, these narratives bear witness to the human spirit's ability to overcome, adjust, and rejoice in triumphantly confronting dermatological obstacles.